QUIT SMOKING FOREVER!

Madison Mason

QUIT SMOKING FOREVER!

Congratulations on buying this book! This is a great moment for you.

If you are a smoker, I predict this will prove to be the most important book you will ever buy. And compared to the benefits you will reap in improved, good health, longer life and more time spent with your loved ones, plus accomplishing the things you want to do in life, one day you'll look on this book as a tiny little bit of money very, very well spent!

Having said that, I have good news and not so good. First the good news.

Once you've read this little book and learned to apply the simple techniques you'll be shown, **YOU WILL QUIT SMOKING FOREVER**. Guaranteed.

The not so good news is: YOU have to do it. No one can do it for you. It's simple, it's easy, but it's going to require commitment and perseverance. You're the one who started smoking; you're the one who will end it.
You **WILL!** I KNOW you can do it. I did it. Others did. So will you.

So once again, Congratulations!

You are ready RIGHT NOW to
QUIT SMOKING FOREVER or you wouldn't even have this book in your hands.
I'm with you. Let's go!

QUIT SMOKING FOREVER!

I admit I'm probably obnoxious to a lot of people.
I'm a crusader. And aren't they annoying?
I go up to total strangers on the street and say
"Hey! Stop smoking that crap!" Actually, more
often I use a much stronger word than crap, but
you get the picture. (On my best behavior here.)
Oh, I say it nicely, I don't yell at them. Still, I
have entered their world without permission.

Some glower, offended at my self righteous
conceit, These turn away mumbling something
I'm glad I don't hear. Others grin sheepishly and
say "Yeah, I know you're right. I'm trying." Then
they suck another lungful. That's how hard
they're trying.

But I don't bug them about it. I've done my job.
The seed's been planted. They've got the thought.
It might flower that day, week, month, or years
from then, but eventually they will make the
attempt to quit smoking that 'crap'. Because I
believe EVERYONE WHO HAS THE HABIT
WANTS TO QUIT. Deep down they really do. But
they feel they can't. And as long as they feel that
way, they're right.

They think they like smoking, for a multitude of reasons which I'll go into later, but if they COULD quit, they WOULD. You may be one of them, I certainly was. For decades. And if you are, when that day comes (and I hope it's today) this little book is here for you.

Because if you follow these simple instructions to the letter YOU **WILL QUIT SMOKING CIGARETTES FOREVER!**
I guarantee it. I did it. And so can you.

If I'm wrong I'll refund your money, no questions asked.
You'll have lost nothing, and you got a free book.
You can keep on smoking and I wish you luck.

But if I'm right, *and **I am**,*

YOU'LL BE FREE!

So let's continue.

A LITTLE TOBACCO HISTORY

I would love to make this book a nice, touchy-feely-comfy experience, but I'm afraid the cold fact is that we're battling an insidious well funded monster, here that masquerades as our friend. It's called Tobacco. Big Tobacco!
It is NOT our friend. It is our ENEMY, and it's been known to be one since its very discovery. And we all-***need***-to be aware of this!

So. Here's a little HISTORY OF TOBACCO.

1492! Columbus sails the ocean blue and is offered dried tobacco leaves as a gift from the "Indians" he met. He thought he was in India. My suspicion?... they were thinking, "Maybe this will kill these guys off and we won't have to." More ships come to "The Indies." Columbus' men get hooked on smoking right off and complain they can't stop. And you can imagine how rough the stuff must have been back then. His sailors start bringing the crap home to make some extra dough, and before long it's grown all over Europe.

Sir Walter Raleigh introduces Virginia tobacco to England in the late 1500s.

Oh boy, Europeans love it! They believe tobacco can cure everything, including, ready for this? Cancer! They also believe that slicing a person's veins open and letting their blood seep out was really good medicine for them, as was introducing maggots and leeches into their bodies. Okay...

So in the 1500s it's the Bitcoin of Europe, everybody's talking about it, using it, buying, selling, trying to cash in. It's even used as money!

Doctors write books lauding the wonderful health benefits of tobacco use. Probably, they were making tons of dough from it. Cured all sorts of ills, didn't it? Today's doctors love prescribing opioids, and they get flown to exotic places for free by their dope dealer pharmo-masters for "conferences."

However, there were early skeptics. The great explorer Sir Francis Bacon complained publicly that it was a nasty habit and very hard to quit.

King James railed against the custom as "lothsome to the eye, hatefull to the Nose, harmefull to the braine, dangerous to the Lungs, and a blacke stinking fume" basically resembling emissions from Hell. Of course, he then imposed a royal monopoly so that he could control all importation and and sales and glom up the pig's portion of the revenue.

Also, guess what else became associated with tobacco. Righty-o! Cancer!   A guy named Tom Harriet, a Virginia settler and grower, dies of nose cancer from snorting snuff and exhaling tobacco smoke through his honker. Must have been a slow, hideous and very unpleasant way to go. And not too great to look at. Sorry about the schnozz, Tom.

When the colonies were well rooted in the "New World" the first black slaves were brought from Africa to grow Tobacco for import. So Tobacco money fueled the enslavement of captive human beings for unpaid labor.

Incidentally, most of the slaves were sent to the Virginia colony. Tobacco shipped to England could, by law, only come from Virginia because, Oh Yeah, it was mostly owned by good King James! First major colony…? You got it, Jamestown! James' Town? The fix was in. Side note: King James later rewarded Sir Walter by chopping his head off. There's gratitude for you.

So you see! Tobacco manufacture had its dark, sinister side even four hundred years ago.

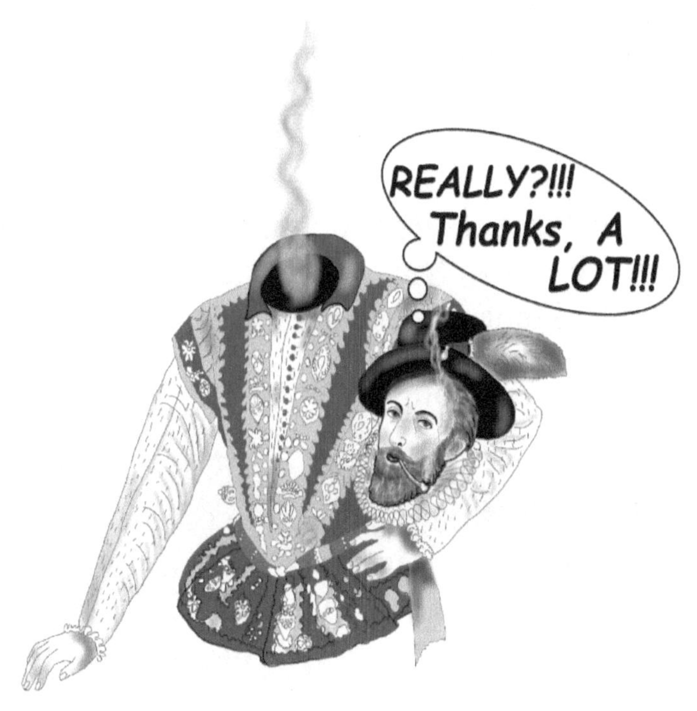

SIR WALLY

(Minus Noggin) c 1618

Ironical, isn't it, that our present physical and psychological slavery was powered for centuries by real human slavery, suffering and deprivation?

The French got theirs brought in through their ambassador Jean Nicot. His stuff was called Nicotiana. Hence, Nicotine?

And Le Beat goes on.

Later, another Frenchman, Pierre Lorillard establishes the first big tobacco company in America, which now is the oldest. Hmm, wonder who picked and hauled and cured all their leaves...? Tobacco = Slavery! I'm just sayin'!

The French introduced it to the Ottoman empire and the Islamic world got hooked, even kids smoked. The Portuguese took it to Japan and Asians have been smoking like chimneys ever since. The Spanish hauled it to Africa and South America and the English got it into Russia. And, naturally, all the monarchs got paid off along the way. Big bucks to be had in killing people. Always.

In the 1800s scientists discovered that 'Nicotine' was the main active and addictive ingredient and also, as it turns out, a deadly poison. The Big T boys and their lawyers have been fighting and refuting this fact ever since.

Then in the 1800s came cigarettes. Up until then consumption had been mainly via pipes, cigars, chews and snuffs. By the early 1900s the tobacco pushers had machined up, and mass production and advertising were nicely combined to hook the entire world on smoking as healthy and fun! Even Ronald Reagan sold coffin nails.

During WWII, Big Tcleverly managed to get their cigarettes packed into the soldiers' ration kits, thereby hooking whole new generations. Maybe those nice men just gave them away for free. Doesn't seem likely though, does it? Wonder whose tax bucks paid the tobacco companies for that?

I remember talking to an old man in England who had been a young soldier in the Dunkirk evacuation. He said the minute they landed back on English soil they were given a blanket, a sandwich and a pack of cigarettes.

And he didn't even smoke. He began that day. Here, kid, try this. You're a soldier! It's manly!

In the 60s Big T got caught admitting they knew they were in the business of making 'nicotine delivery systems', no more, no less. Oh yeah, they also realized their future lay in getting it to kids aged 13 to 18. Their studies told them once they got those babies hooked they pretty much had them for life.   Cough Cough!   Ka-ching, ka-ching.

So, as you go through this little life saver book, keep all the above in mind.

Life is beautiful. I want to save yours and get your health to its optimum!

That's my goal.

ADDICTION

Hey! That's a nasty habit!
How many times have we heard that? From smokers and non-smokers alike. Even my dad told me that once, as he fired up a cancer stick. "Don't ever start this, it's a nasty habit," he coughed. Everybody agrees.

But what does 'nasty' mean? Nasty as in dirty? Ashes and cigarette butts everywhere? Discarded packs and boxes lying on the streets in the rain?

Or nasty as in it stinks? You know somebody's smoking around the corner and a hundred feet away. Even smokers don't like walking into a smoke filled room or bar at first. Takes a little getting used to. It's an acrid, offensive odor that repels, yet clings. You can feel your air being cut off.

To me, the nastiest part of the smoking habit are the rituals behind the addiction that decorate and inform every move we make. Now the habit becomes an insidious, three pronged affair operating on separate levels.

Prong one; the drug addiction. Nicotine is a seriously addictive drug. I've known junkies who kicked years of heroin and/or crack addiction, but can't stop smoking cigarettes. And they're legal and available everywhere.

Prong two; and probably the one that gets us into smoking initially, is the psychological habit of thinking we're cool. We're adult, daring, outsiders. We're cavalier, living on the edge. Other people don't get it. We're a club. We understand each other. We share!

Prong three; the physical component. What we do with our hands, our fingers, our mouths. There's a whole dance involved. Everybody's got their own style. We pick up neat tricks from other cool people.

PRONG ONE — Nicotine Addiction

Oddly, this is probably the easiest part to quit. There are patches, pills, supplements that can provide the drug. But it's addictive and deadly. Hey, it's used as pesticide. Who doesn't want pesticide in their blood stream? If it's so good for butterflies and bees it's got to be good for us! *...Yeah...*

The fact is, when you quit, your body begins immediately repairing itself. Isn't that beautiful? It starts sloughing off toxins right away. Actually it's been doing it all along but you're not giving it a chance to catch up.
Drink plenty of water. Exercise regularly, sweat it out. And make sure you supply the body with Vitamin C, either as a supplement or in Citrus Juice.
The physical addiction falls away within a day or two, then fades quickly.

Your blood pressure, heart rate and adrenaline levels return to normal, constriction in your veins, arteries and blood vessels shrinks, nerve endings begin repairing themselves, appetite returns and hey, you just feel better!
Nothing wrong with that!

PRONG TWO — The Cool Factor

Okay, who can ever get over the image of cool James Dean, hair rumpled, collar turned up, gazing dreamily off camera with a cigarette dangling from his lips? Not me. That's the mind picture that legitimized smoking to me. So cool.

That pose has been repeated countless times in our advertising zeitgeist on a second rate level because it's totally iconic. But it's a ***pose***, that's all! There are a dozen different shots of him, always ***same pose***. Now that's selling, folks.

Or how about Bette Davis and her sexy hauteur in, well, any movie, cigarette in hand and smoke emanating from every facial orifice? She was the epitome of cool self assurance. And she made smoking an art. No wonder they paid her big bucks to put her face in Chesterfield ads. Also Lucky Strike bought her for a testimonial ad touting mildness on the throat. That lady could smoke! I actually used to practice smoking like Bette.
More on what smoking did to her later.

Well sorry, it's not cool, and increasingly less so. Period. As smokers, we're looked on more and more as social pariahs, delusional losers. Death wish dummies. Lung junkies! We know it, we sense it and yet...
Did I say insidious?

PRONG THREE — The dance

The coffee, the cocktail, the after-the-meal smoke. The fingers, the hands, the lips. The French inhale, smoke rings, the lip grip, the dangle, the tap, crush, flip, the stomp. All the comfortable steps we memorize in the slow, smoky dance of death. Because that's what it is. We get tired of it, we get bored with it, yet we dance on.

I'm going to give you a nice easy new habit replace all those steps and get your breathing back to normal. Just keep reading.

BRAIN WASHING

For years, since the beginning of movies, the powers that be have clearly understood the hypnotic value of cinema. If a picture's worth a thousand words, a 'Moving' picture is worth a million bucks. You get a bunch of people sitting in a dark room watching other people, who they think are more interesting and glamorous than they are, and doing things that they don't do, those folks are going to emulate that behavior. Plain and simple.
Hitler's guys knew this better than anyone. Look at Nazi propaganda films.

So it didn't take long for the tobacco boys to realize the possibilities and rush to plant the power of the smoking image in movies. Money changed hands, the big Muckers in Hollywood took the dough behind the scenes, and Lo and Behold! The screen became clouded with tobacco smoke.

I love the old classic movies. Grew up on them. I watch them now and I realize how many people smoked, or pretended to smoke in the movies we loved. Was there ever a scene where Humphrey Bogart wasn't puffing on a gasper? He even pitched woo to Lauren Bacall while burning cigarettes. Nothing sexier than the two of them firing it up over hot eyeballs.

As I said, Bette Davis made smoking an art to be practiced. It became elegant, sophisticated, arch, and even catty. She made it sharp or languid, depending on her mood. She would even take a puff and let the smoke run from her mouth up into her nostrils, the old "French inhale."
Don't think I didn't practice that one in front of the mirror just to look cool.

It's tragic, but dozens, perhaps hundreds of great actors and other notables have died of ugly, agonizing diseases related to years of smoking.
And many of them, far too young.
I could list them here but it goes on forever.
Are you interested? It's all on the web.

I said earlier I'd tell you why I was crusader.
Okay, this is one of my primary reasons. Patrick Swayze was a dear friend of mine. And I'm sure we all agree, never was there a more beautiful young man. He'd been a heavy smoker his whole life. As you probably know, he died much too young and way before his time of pancreatic cancer. I saw Patrick just before he passed away.

He was ravaged by the disease, gaunt, drawn, and in constant suffering. He was spending hundreds of thousands just to stay alive a little bit longer. He had wasted away to about 125 pounds by my estimation, but still tough in his jeans and boots as we were walking around his corral jawboning, for what we both knew was the last time. It was a painful scene and we were talking heart to heart. He knew he was going and it wouldn't be long. I was holding back tears when he suddenly pulled out a cigarette and lit it up. I was legitimately shocked! I said "Buddy, what the hell are you doing? Are you crazy?" He snorted and replied, "What? You afraid it's going to give me cancer?"

I had no reply. It was classic gallows humor, but he had a point. The damage was done. It was all over. He was losing everything. Lisa, the ranch, the horses, the career, his life. What would be the purpose of stopping then? But I loved that guy, and I miss him, and I will as long as I live. And I lament at how much he more could have done with a few added healthy years.

I only tell this story to illustrate that I understand how hard it can be to quit this insidious slavery.

Desi Arnaz, America's favorite Cuban and Lucy's beleaguered husband, the beloved Ricky Ricardo,

died early of horrible smoking related diseases.
In his last days he launched a haunting video on
YouTube. He was gaunt, hollow, could barely
breathe and pleaded with his audience "Never
ever start smoking".
I can't find that video any more. Seems that
someone in power pulled it. Gee…who do ya
think?…
Desi and Lucy Jr, on losing their father, also
posted their own anti smoking video, again, it's
also been yanked from YouTube and gone like a
puff of…smoke.
Oh my, wonder who managed that one?
But in a sick, twisted irony, YouTube allows the
video of the old cigarette commercial Light one
Up For Lucy to play on.
I seem to remember this clearly. Maybe I'm
wrong, but I don't think so.

But if Big Tobacco can keep a strangle hold on
your elected officials, stifling information on
Google should be no problem. It's all about
throwing money in the right faces. They know
that, Been doing it for a century or more.

Now Voyager is a 40s classic, a romantic pot
boiler of a film starring Bette Davis and Paul
Henreid. She's the deeply troubled, rich ugly

duckling who becomes a gorgeous swan and he's the elegant, suave, but deeply troubled European who helps her emerge. And believe it or not, they fall in love! It's a great, classic movie and one of the best cigarette commercials ever. They smoke so much that everyone on the set must have been choking. He pulls the iconic move of lighting two cigarettes at the same time. His and Hers, how cool is that? He gives her one, for which she gazes gratefully and lovingly into his eyes.

But here's the final kicker, as if we, the audience, aren't already hooked. In the last scene, with violins trembling, they find each other again, but realize their love will never work and they must nobly part.

But instead of a last embrace, a soft kiss, champagne toast, an "I love you," Handsome Paul gazes deep into the eyes of Dreamy Bette and actually says, to her...

"Let's have a cigarette on it." Ka-Ching!!

Well you can bet the audience wasn't even out of the lobby before they were digging in their pockets and their purses for a smoke or heading to the drugstore to take up the habit. How's that for planting a brain bomb? Butt sales must have tripled in 1943!

By the way, Bogie, our brilliant and iconic
Humphrey Bogart succumbed to smoking related
cancer of the esophagus at the ripe old age of 56.
R.I.P.
Bette Davis suffered cancer and stroke.
Glamorous.

Sorry, Carry on...

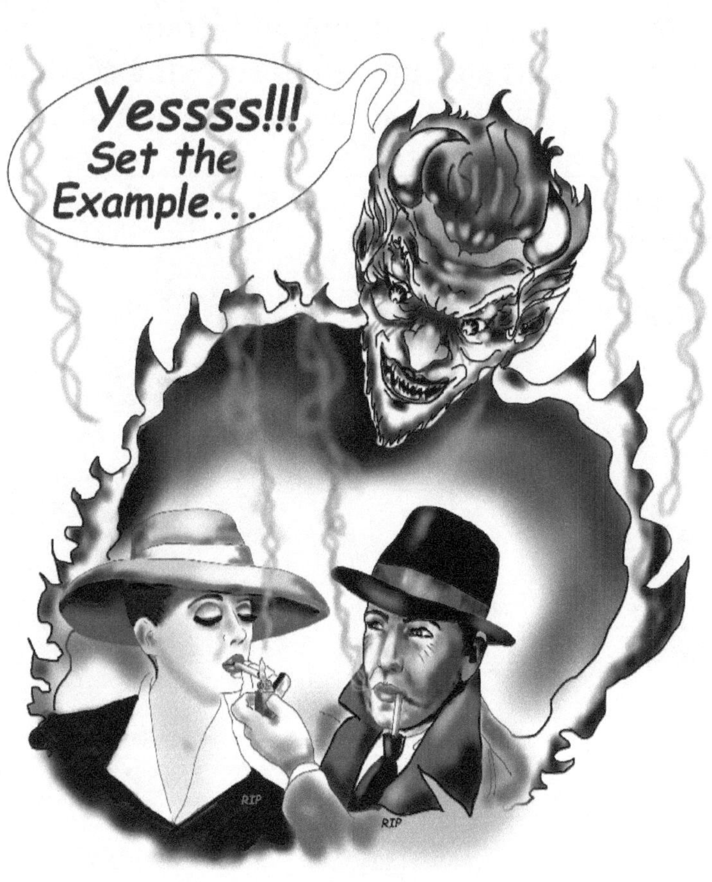

OUR HEROES!

MODELED BEHAVIOR

Both of my parents smoked. I watched them as a child, my exemplars, and thought how grand and controlled they were, each handling the mystical ceremony of the cigarette in their own way, having their coffee or cocktail. Or just smoking for no reason whenever they wanted.
Because they could.
I thought it was a thing they chose to do. How could I know they were addicted to tobacco for life and couldn't stop? But I do remember their saying occasionally that they wished they'd never started. Now that I recall, they smoked in bed just before going to sleep and fired one up first thing in the morning, usually with coffee. Coffee and a cigarette, the two wheels of the morning bicycle to hell.

My dad's style was dramatic and masculine. He would pull the pack of Chesterfields from his shirt pocket, jog it slightly so just one cigarette would pop up, raise the pack to his lips, gently roll the white cylinder over the tip of his tongue to dampen it. He'd pull out his silver Zippo, open it with the trademark clank, and spin the striker wheel with that classic Zippo sound. The lighter fluid whoofed into blue and yellow flame and you could hear the paper and shredded tobacco catch fire. He'd take a deep draw as he clacked the cover shut and replaced the lighter. Then he'd pull the cigarette from his mouth and exhale for what seemed like a count of ten. Later, when he'd smoked it down to a stub, dangerously close to his lip, talking with it bouncing up and down as the smoke burned his left eye, with one hissing intake he would take the last quick drag and flip the butt forcefully into the air, to burn out, who knows where. The smoke softly whooshed from his mouth in focused stream, dissipated, and vanished forever. Naturally, I wanted to be a heroic figure like that guy one day. Little did I know.

My mother, a fine, well bred Southern lady, had a much more elegant style about her. She would delicately touch the flame to the tip of her Kool cigarette as she looked down her nose, take a quick, delicate puff, inhale briefly, while her hand assumed a regal position off to the side of her face, pointing upwards, several inches from her cheek, fingers arched in a dancer's pose, at the ready. Before each gentle puff she would softly tap the cylinder over an ashtray with a manicured finger, so no ash would drop accidentally on her lovely protruding bosom.

Outside, of course, she would never be so crude as to callously flip her cigarette away, but dropped her unwanted remains straight down and gently ground it underfoot with feminine finality.
Too girly a style for me. I was destined to be a manly butt flipper.

I was a kid in North Carolina. They grow and manufacture the stuff there. It's a major force in the economy. If you don't smoke they ask you to move to another state. I was smoking as a nine year old. I bought them as a child and it seemed okay with everyone. Lucky Strikes, their trademark bright red ball. Ooooooh, Red! In my childhood a pack cost fifteen cents to a quarter. The really harsh ones the old farmers smoked, called Picayunes or Fatimas, cost a dime a pack. Real coffin nails. A drag off one of those was like inhaling a basketball. It hurt. But that didn't stop me.

My dad let me smoke one of his Camels at the age of nine and had a hearty laugh as I choked and coughed. He thought he was dissuading me, but little did he know that he was really accepting me and validating me as a man.

My mom forbade my smoking, so naturally I
stole hers when she wasn't looking. She thought
smoking mentholated cigarettes was better for
her. I hated the taste and the effect of all those
added chemicals. I really couldn't stand them,
but that sure didn't deter me. Neither did
coughing, choking, dizziness or puking.
Learning to smoke was not easy or pleasant.
What could have made me so determined?
Advertising?

I remember being taken on an all day field trip in
the eighth grade. How exciting! Dress nicely and
get to school early. Busses are waiting. Where
are we going? The class is going to visit the RJ
Reynolds Tobacco Factory in Winston Salem!
Oh wow! RJ Reynolds!

So we arrive in Winston Salem after a couple
hours and lunch on the way. Our bus pulls up in
front of the beautiful, modern aluminum and
glass offices of The RJ Reynolds Tobacco
Company! We climb out of the bus and tromp
inside. What a delight for goggle eyed kids!
There, in the center of a brightly lit, terrazzo
floored lobby stands a gigantic statue of a
CAMEL, (Camel Cigarettes, remember?) made
entirely of shredded tobacco! Of course it's the

coolest thing any of us nose pickers have ever
laid eyes on.
Then we're given a tour of the super - factory.
We watch them separate the leaves, chop them,
shred the tobacco and roll, cut and pack
thousands of cigarettes in bright white paper at
lightning speed. It's amazing! And our tour guide
is a sweet, soft, drawling beauty queen right off
the pages of a magazine cigarette ad.
A teenage boy's dream! I'm in heaven. I'm in the
holy of holies, RJ Reynolds! I'm *in*!

Then, to show us how much they like us, and
respect us as future smokers, we are given *free*
packs of cigarettes as we leave! Winstons, or
Salems, depending on your preference. But these
are really cool ones you can't get in the stores,
five smokes to a pack. In little flip boxes. And, get
this, they like us! So we can take as many of
them as we want!
Free! No limit! They like us!
I ride happily back home with my pockets
packed. My future is assured!

Soon I work my way through the sick, dizzy,
coughing and throwing up stage and persevere
until I'm a solid citizen smoker. More than that,
I'm a proud smoker, a very cool guy. Not a kid

anymore, I'm a real James Dean wannabe badass. At fifteen I'm buying my own on a regular basis.

I notice I can't run as fast or far any more. I' m out of breath easily. I have a dry mouth and throat. Stinky breath. Tan teeth. But I persevere.
        Hey, I've been to RJ Reynolds! None of you guys have. They like me! I'm special!

A lot of the other kids rolled their pack in their tee shirt sleeve. I didn't care for that. it looked cool, but it smashed the smokes. And they were precious.
Also, that made them too obvious. We weren't really supposed to be doing it. But if you were caught, you just told the teacher you were holding them for somebody else. For some baffling reason that always seemed to work.

So now, at 16, I have a solid pack a day habit.
A two pack a day habit at 18.
A steady, enduring habit for 20 years.
A heart attack at 48. Down for the count and on my way out.

WHAT SMOKING DOES TO YOU

Sorry, everyone. I warned you this would not be a soft, fuzzy piece of work. I'm not purposely trying to scare you, but we smokers are battling a tough, devious enemy who has one intention only and it's not in our best interests.

So, briefly, this is what modern medicine knows smoking does to you. Smoking tobacco attacks virtually every single organ in your body.

It causes, for sure, without any doubt:
Cancer
Stroke
Heart attack
Emphysema
Vascular Disease
Chronic Pulmonary Obstructive Disease
Heart Disease
Asthma
And a bunch more

Any of these appeal to you? No!

So we're going to get you off this garbage, once and for all!
Come with me.

By the way, a brief moment of confession here.
I'm strong and healthy, thank Heaven. I work
out, run, take tap dance and hip hop classes and
can give you thirty push ups even at my
frighteningly advanced age. But I had a big ass
heart attack in 1991 and was flat on my back in
Cedars Sinai with a dozen very worried looking
professionals standing around, their machines
humming, beeping with colored lights flashing.
They didn't know whether I would stay or go. I
made it, thanks to deft work by a terrific
cardiologist, Dr. Norman Lepor with whom I'm
still great pals. But I was in very good shape then
and couldn't figure out why this had happened to
me, since I didn't seem to fit the paradigm; not
overweight, not out of shape, didn't live on
greasy fast food, heavy booze or illegal drugs,
why me? A doctor asked me if I had ever
smoked. Sure, I said, for a couple decades or
more. She told me it was the absolute worst thing
you can do to your body, and went on to list all
the nasty work tobacco smoking inflicts on your
soft and vulnerable internal system. I had quit at
that point for about five years but she said the
damage had been done long, long ago.
I was shocked.

Anyway, you don't need that. So let's get you off
these things. Now!
Moving along...

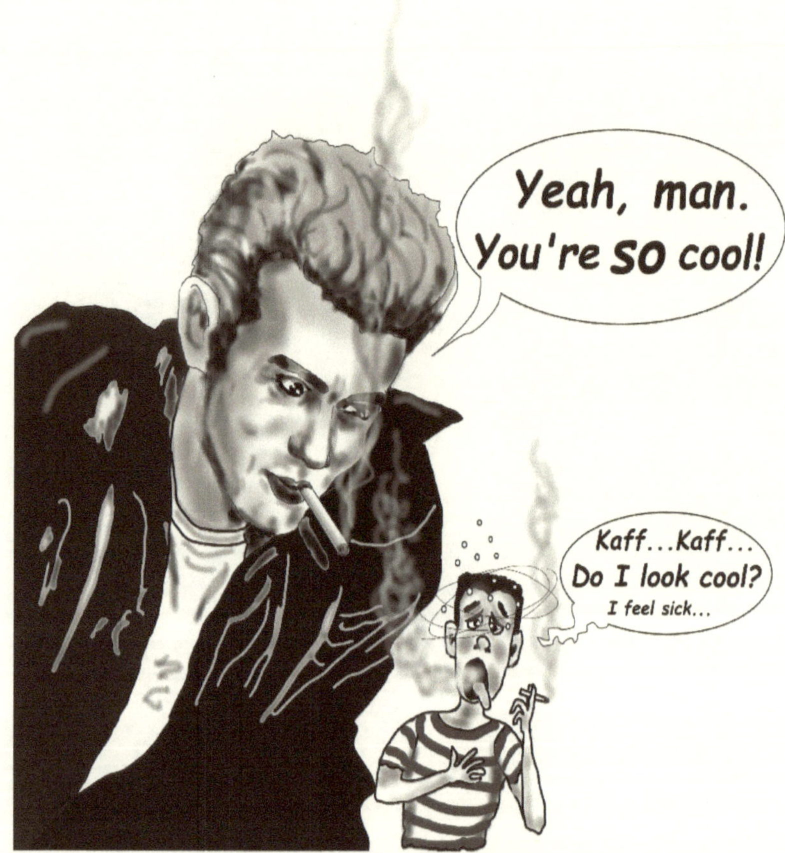

SOOO COOOL!!!!!

CORPO-**RAT**-IONS

The Tobacco Industry, like so many other
businesses that only bode ill for mankind, is
deeply entrenched in the real business of making,
what?...
Right, money.
They exist for no other reason.
Are they evil men and women? No.
Or...probably not.
Do they really care if you live or die? No. Not
really.
Do they care if you use their product and feed
their bottom line? Oh, You bet!

Same as the makers of assault weapons, designed
for the sole purpose of killing other human
beings. They're doing it for the MONEY!
I call these people CORPO-**RATS**.

They hire and surround themselves with gangs of
lawyers. These legal-thug-body guards are paid
to protect the corpo-rats from you, should
anything go wrong. They *also* don't care about
you on any kind of human or moral level. It's
about the bucks, plain and simple.
And yet *you're* the person who's actually paying
their fees! Ironical, no?

There's something so twisted in all this.

So the corpo-rats spend tons of dollars and hire big experts and have endless meetings around conference tables to examine what their product is, what it does, how it can be improved, updated, more effectively disseminated, how they can get it into the kids, and what their liabilities are.

They know very well what tobacco does to people. They are fully aware of the disastrous effects of long term use on the human body. At this point in history, nobody's got their head in the sand on this. Volumes of scientific studies and reports have been written. It' s all common knowledge.

And yet, they keep planting it, developing it, nurturing it, harvesting it, manufacturing, and marketing it.

And they've never been included in The War On Drugs.

And the politicians you vote for and elect to protect you - simply look the other way. With their hands out.
Sick.

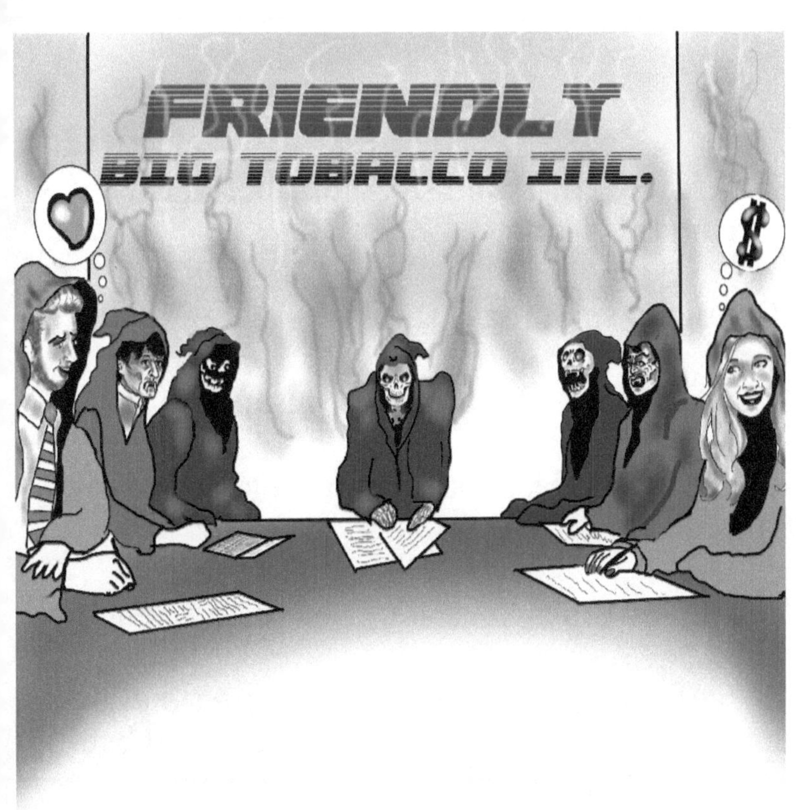

EXCUSE ME...
FRIENDS OF YOURS?

DO IT NOW!

The great Mark Twain said, long before any of us
were on this planet;

"Giving up smoking is the easiest thing in the
world.
I know because I've done it thousands of times."

Wry humor indeed, but so apt. It's Mark Twain,
after all.

How many times have you tried to quit...and
failed?
Me? At least a dozen, probably more times over
the years. And still I eventually wandered back.
And it always started with just one cigarette.
Just one.
Truth, I didn't like that one very much. But I did
it anyway.

That tells me that my low lying, subconscious
addiction was ever alert, even though I hadn't
smoked for months, maybe even years,
depending.

So here's how my progression went. See if this is familiar.

I decide to quit. Good!
But I think about it... I waffle... And I smoke.
Then I realize I've failed. Oooh. Lousy feeling.
I get angry and throw away the pack.
Now it's done. No more! I turn my back and it's over.
But is it? Of course not. We know that,
I make it though the first couple withdrawal days.
Lots of gum. The monkey won't stop chattering. Calling me.
Coffee in the mornings is rough. So is cocktail time.
But I make it! Yay Me!

Now the monkey starts to settle down and leave me alone.
I start to feel good about myself. My great accomplishment!
I hang tough. I brag.
I stay out of smoky places. The urge subsides over the next three weeks.
I'm home free! Yay Me again! I quit smoking!
Time goes by, a few months, a year, maybe two, I don't think about it.

I feel so much better. I can breathe. No chest pain.
Food tastes great.
I'm a renewed Human Being! Fresh and healthy.
Then I wind up at a party. Couple drinks.
Someone lights up. Want one?
Umm...sure, thanks. Uh oh...
Come on...I can do just one...
Maybe another one. Now I'm smoking!
Hey, can I bum a smoke? Hey, you mind if I...?
After a few days of this I get tired of feeling like a bum.
Sure, people give over, but they have this look in their eye.
I'll buy my own pack. Just have maybe, one smoke a day. That'll last 20 days. Good!
Yep. You know the routine. All gone the next day. Or two. All smoked up.
Aw man!...
Okay, buy another pack. I'll stash it away. Make this one last.
Right, maybe I make it three quarters of a day on this pack.
Now I'm on the ride and securely strapped in.
I'm a smoker! Again!

But here's the truth. Not really again... ***Still!***

The Demon was hiding in there the whole time waiting to jump me and take me down. And I gave him a key and the free pass to do it!
Why?!!!
Because somewhere deep down inside, there was still lurking the **DESIRE**!
I'd quit the habit, but I never killed the habitué. The old desire. The want! It'd been skulking the whole time.
It never went away, or I wouldn't have done it again. If I didn't want it, I wouldn't have done it, right? It was so subtle, so hidden, but obviously, it was *always* alert.
I had the **desire** to do it!

My theory is once you started smoking; from that day on you're a smoker.
You're either a smoker who's smoking or a smoker who's not smoking.
But I found a way to ***kill that Demon for good!***

So we're going to get you to quit smoking.
You and I.
And we're going to do it by getting rid of the desire.

You can **DO IT!**

Say **YES I CAN!**

<u>Say</u> it!

YES I *CAN!*

GOOD FOR YOU!

THE TECHNIQUE

You want to **QUIT SMOKING FOREVER** and you're ready, or you wouldn't have bought this book.

THIS IS THE TIME for you to **STOP!**

YOU HAVE CHOSEN this time. Way to go!

No matter where you are in life it is never too late. This is the beginning of your new life of **HEALTH, STRENGTH** and **FREEDOM!**

I have written those words in bold caps to point out that this is about your **thinking**. Not chemicals, but **thoughts**. And this may come as a great big surprise to some people, but you can control your thoughts. In fact the key to power is the control of thought. Think about it for a minute.

I'll give you an example of how to control your thoughts.

Look at your hand. Really look at it. Stare at it. Count to ten, nice and slow.

Notice the different colors in your hand.
Look at the subtle pinks and blues.
Notice the veins.
Notice the lines.
Look at the shadows.
Look at the highlights
Look at all the subtle curves
Close the hand slightly.
Now look at your nails.
See at how everything changes when you move just slightly.

Okay, that's enough. Let's not obsess on hands here. We could go on forever. The point is you started with just a hand, and by controlling your thoughts you had a dozen different experiences. In less than a minute.

If you actually did the above exercise I can tell you, you did great! Now you see what your thoughts can do. And this is how you're going to **QUIT SMOKING FOREVER!**

You've probably heard this a hundred times; to break a habit we have to replace it with another habit. That's because it's true. It's all in our mind!

The habit we're going to replace is simply a habit of **YOUR THOUGHT!** Studies reveal that we have 50,000 thoughts in a single day. We're just going to control **(1)** one of them.
Smoking, as a habit, has become unconscious. Automatic. You get the urge. There's your **thought**. The routine kicks in. Another **thought.** It may be all unconscious to a great degree, but you drive another nail into the coffin. We're going to change that, and it's easy. You've made the decision to turn your back on cigarettes FOREVER! It's over! So here's what you do.

Now please, **MEMORIZE** the these *eight simple words*:

**I HAVE LOST
ALL DESIRE
TO SMOKE CIGARETTES**

Say them softly to yourself. Good.
Say them again.
Say them once more. Now, four times!
Excellent! We're on the path!

Congratulations again! You decided you want to quit smoking and that's why you bought this book, maybe the most important and honest

words you'll ever read. But just owning these
pages does not guarantee you will

QUIT SMOKING FOREVER!

Only by **true dedication** to your good health;
only by **diligent,** and real, **determined
application of the simple techniques** you'll
learn here, will you be free from tobacco forever.
We want determination.
DE-TERMINATION.
Determination = A firm or fixed intention to
achieve a desired end.
One of those wonderful combo words that
comprise the English language.
<u>De</u> = do the opposite of. <u>Termination</u> - end in
time or existence.

So we **NEVER TERMINATE!** Once we make
this decision and commitment to save our health
and prolong our life, (the most important life of
any us will ever know, because without it, how
we can help anyone else?) we
NEVER BACK OFF!

Say out loud, **I CAN DO IT!**   Good for you!

Now, take the thumbnail and the middle
fingernail of each hand and gently squeeze each
earlobe until you can feel the pinch. Like a little
health spider crawling up each ear, go up the
outside edge of the ear to the top and back down
again, feeling that slight pinch as you go. Don't
do it to the point of pain, we're not here to hurt
ourselves, just to stimulate the edge of the ears.
(These are the points acupuncturists would use.)

Repeat: **I HAVE LOST
                      ALL DESIRE
              TO SMOKE CIGARETTES!**

We say this aloud **Twelve Times** while we do
the ear pinching drill.
You can do four sets of three, three sets of four,
two sets of six, whatever makes it easy for you. It
doesn't matter.

What matters is **only** that you:

**DO THIS, INSTEAD OF SMOKING
EVERY TIME YOU FEEL THE URGE
EVERY - SINGLE - TIME**

YOU WILL BE SUCCESSFUL if...

you **ADHERE RELENTLESSLY** to this technique. As relentlessly as you pursued the smoking of tobacco.

Whisper or shout it! Whatever you want to do.
Whatever fits the situation.
Walk away from other people if you have to, if you're embarrassed or want it to be a personal thing, it's cool. This technique will overpower the urge.

I HAVE LOST
ALL DESIRE
TO SMOKE CIGARETTES!

THIS WILL BECOME YOUR TRUTH.

YOU **CAN** MAKE IT!

All you do is apply this technique <u>relentlessly</u>.

BE RELENTLESS!

Remember...

<u>Relentless</u> = No abatement of intensity, strength, or pace!

We **NEVER BACK OFF**, give in, or give up,
NEVER!
No matter what anybody says or does!

WE NEVER SMOKE AGAIN!

YOU NEVER SMOKE AGAIN!

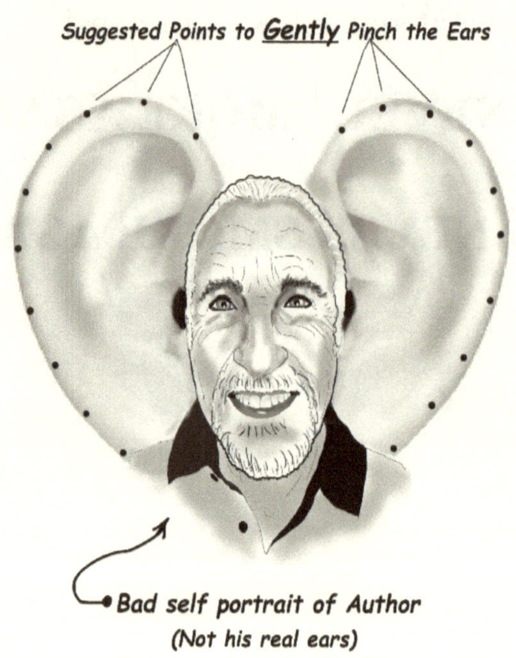

Silly guy, I know.
But it makes the point.

THE NEW YOU

So! This is it! This is your **NEW THINK**. The **NEW HABIT**. This drill, this simple replacement habit will create the new vision, the new person,

THE NEW, HEALTHIER SMOKE FREE YOU!

We're fighting a battle. A battle against a massive, greedy, wealthy, and highly organized enemy who enlists **YOUR** politicians to help them attack you, your health, and your body. They emplo firms of highly paid professional liars and manipulators to take any advantage of you that they can. They've lured you into this deadly habit somehow. And if you suffer or die from using their products and seek redress, they are set up to destroy you by any litigious means they can devise. And they have very deep pockets.

NOW YOU DECLARE WAR!

You do not capitulate or comply with these guys, or cave in! **NEVER!**

You are stronger than they are, because...

YOU CAN SAY NO!

They can't force you to smoke! They haven't
managed to get laws passed requiring you to
smoke. Yet! Your defense against them is to
TURN YOUR BACK.
Cut them out. Cut them off. Dump them!
It's as simple as that.

I'm not on a white horse, nor am I wearing shiny
silver armor, but I am here to save you. I'm here
to protect your life from dark forces
masquerading as your friends. No kidding.
Consider these people your secret enemies.
They've declared war on you. I mean it. It;s
about money to them.
They have long meetings around conference
tables to determine the best way to hook you on
their addictive products and destroy your health.
They know perfectly damn well what their stuff
does. But it's all about getting you to give them
your money.
Billboards? Completely ignore them. Look away.
See an ad with smiley models showing you how
happy they are to be flirting with cancer and
vascular disease? Posers getting paid. Tear up the

ads and throw them away. And utter a curse on them as you do. Fight back!
Then take a deep breath of fresh air and meditate on how good it feels to be alive and free. It's great!

Be HAPPY!

Indulge in your new habit!
EVERY TIME you feel the urge for a cigarette, **INSTEAD OF SMOKING,** do your drill! Like a soldier. Like the guardian of your life. Pinch the earlobes a dozen times, repeat softly a dozen times those beautiful, and empowering words. Your Declaration of Independence!

Say them again now! Your eternal affirmation. Your mantra for life. . .

I HAVE LOST
ALL DESIRE
TO SMOKE CIGARETTES!
I HAVE LOST
ALL DESIRE
TO SMOKE CIGARETTES!

I HAVE LOST
ALL DESIRE
TO SMOKE CIGARETTES!
I HAVE LOST
ALL DESIRE
TO SMOKE CIGARETTES!

I HAVE LOST
ALL DESIRE
TO SMOKE CIGARETTES!
I HAVE LOST
ALL DESIRE
TO SMOKE CIGARETTES!

I HAVE LOST
ALL DESIRE
TO SMOKE CIGARETTES!
I HAVE LOST
ALL DESIRE
TO SMOKE CIGARETTES!

I HAVE LOST
ALL DESIRE
TO SMOKE CIGARETTES!
I HAVE LOST
ALL DESIRE
TO SMOKE CIGARETTES!

I HAVE LOST
ALL DESIRE
TO SMOKE CIGARETTES!
I HAVE LOST
ALL DESIRE
TO SMOKE CIGARETTES!

Make these words your dependable habit and you will never smoke again!

It may be a little tough at first. There is no easy way out. I wish there was. Sorry. It took your will power to get into it, it'll take your **won't** power to get out of it. Wish I could make it soft and cuddly for you. I just can't.
You have to soldier up. You have made the decision! You turned your back, and now you have the tools. **Do it! Every time!** And believe! This works! **Do it!**
I know you can! I've seen it work.
I have faith in you, now you have faith.

Sure, it's hard for a couple days, but not as rough as years on oxygen slowly succumbing to hideous pulmonary diseases.

And the rewards you receive later, the money you save, the way you feel, will more than make up for some little bit of discomfort in the beginning.

And you'll be living a healthy, smoke free life!

YOU CAN DO IT!

<u>NEVER</u> GIVE UP!

END NOTE

Cigarette smoking kills nearly half a million people every year in the U.S. alone. Around the world, its total each year is six million people dead! Every year.
I don't want you or anyone you love to be in that statistic.

And hey! **Cigarette smokers stink!** Come on, I'm not being mean, you know they do! It makes your teeth and eyes yellow. It makes your skin sallow and dried out. If you're smoking, your clothes stink, your hair stinks, your breath, and even your skin. Don't believe me? Smoke a cigarette and hug a little kid, see what they say. They'll tell you exactly where you stand.

Smokers spread their pollution around themselves for hundreds of feet away. How often are you somewhere, and you smell the acrid stench of a burning cigarette? You can't locate where it's coming from but someone is smoking and everybody's having to inhale it. It reeks, it ages you and it kills.

Be a thinker, not a stinker!

On a three hour layover at an airport I noticed they had built a glassed-in garden area for people to escape the synthetic airport environment and get some fresh air. It was a lovely park-like space filled with plants and sunlight. I went in to breathe real air for a while. Oh Mama, Big Mistake. I was walking into living ashtray. The rancid clinging stench from the lung suckers desperate for a jolt, made this oasis uninhabitable. I risked first stage cancer from second stage smoke by just sticking my head in the door. And everyone looked so furtive and guilty, like they knew what they were doing was just all wrong. They all had the look of dogs who had done something on the carpet and got yelled at.
And they sure s hell weren't having any fun. I got out.

As of this writing, a pack of cigarettes in London costs ten British pounds.
That's about fourteen American dollars.
Someone with a two pack a day habit is spending over ten grand a year to kill themselves. Are you kidding?
Does this make any logical sense? No No No! It's the worst kind of consumer slavery.

I want the best for you! No more slavery! No more being a lung junkie! Be smart.

BE FREE!

QUIT SMOKING

FOREVER!

I *know* you can.

Madison Mason